Be Serious about B. Cereus

Enhancing Your Food Handling Practices for Safety and Health

The fate of a nation rides on the health of its people.

Author: Wesley J Allen

Published by: Artistic Word Creations

Contents

Introduction

Many women and men work in the kitchen and do their best for their families and for themselves. Some of these cooks and bakers are very sensitive about their abilities with food. Some are using cultural practices that have been in their families for generations. That makes them very partial to family traditions and, in some cases, unwilling to change what has been handed down to them. They understandably want to honor their ancestors.

It is not a shameful thing to update your food handling strategies. Grandma would be proud that you are keeping up with the times and growing admirably in your position. I hope you will take heed to the strategies expressed in this document. Use what works for you. Take what you like and leave the rest. And most importantly, share what you learn with others.

• • •

This book is about enhancing your food handling practices to avoid the pain and misery that can come from foodborne illnesses.

The Bible says, "For this reason many among you are weak and sick, and a number sleep." That is in reference to the Lord's Supper; but it is not confined to that. It is a spiritual principle. Those who do not take spiritual advice seriously are causing sickness and pain in their lives. They are sleeping spiritually.

Those who will not listen to good sound advice, harm themselves and others. If you commit to enhancing your food handling practices, you can avoid being weak and sick and sleepy.

This book will focus on a bacteria called Bacillus Cereus. What is it? Where does it come from? What can it do to your body? How can you avoid it? How can you get rid of it, if it has already made its home in your body.

• • •

I am writing this book because B. Cereus has already affected my life and the lives of others whom I love. I have witnessed firsthand some of what B. Cereus can do. I have experienced the smell of food with B. Cereus rapidly multiplying in it and creating its toxins. I am writing this book because I was informed about Bacillus Cereus in a dream and admonished to share the information.

• • •

Prior to having the dream, I knew nothing about B. Cereus. The dream prompted me to research it and shed some light on the mystery. I have more than eighty pages of information from AI research. The information comes from our Intelligence which fills cyberspace. I love Meta and Gemini. They may be robots, but they don't speak from their own minds. They gather, in seconds, the pertinent information from reputable sources. The National Institutes of Health- NIH, Penn Medicine, and the United Nations Office for Project Services – UNOPS are among the sources of the information gathered here.

• • •

It is my hope that this book will help many people out of some of the physical pains and misery of life, to which we subject ourselves, because of lack of knowledge. All my life I have heard the cliché – "What you don't know won't hurt you." On the contrary, what you don't know can disable or kill you at the worst; and at the least can make your life miserable.

It is my hope that this book will reach the innocent minds of those who act on cultural beliefs and traditions and are hurting themselves and others because of a learned food handing practice handed down to them.

It is my hope that whole communities and even countries of people will learn to Be Serious about B. Cereus and will better their lives due to less disease and pain at the dispelling of ignorance about simple food handling practices.

It is my hope that you will read this book and pass the newly gained knowledge on to many more who can be helped by it.

It is my hope that some of the diseases that are claimed to have unknown causes and cures will mysteriously disappear from the lives of those they affect.

It is my hope that everything I write here will honor God and that the food handling practices we adopt will be honorable to God and all who come to our tables to eat.

The fate of a nation rides on the health of its people.

Chapter 1-This'll Be My Home

Now, the Boll Weevil was a little black bug, come from Mexico they say, ah hanh, come all the way to Texas, just a looking for a place to stay. Just a looking for a home. Just looking for a home.

Some may still have trouble with bugs in the flour or bugs in the grain; but they are not nearly as harmful as the bacteria that makes its home in your food. Bugs do bring in impurities and bacteria of their own; but they can be kept out of the food easily enough with the use of closed storage containers. However, many foods naturally contain microorganisms including bacteria, yeast, and mold. Some bacteria are harmless or even beneficial, while others cause foodborne illnesses.

Bacterium comes from the earth. Way back in The Garden of Eden, because two people didn't listen to spiritual advice, God cursed the ground upon which we stand. Afterwards it brought forth thorns and thistles. It must be cultivated to remove stones and roots and bugs and worms, and the soil must be fertilized. Pesticides must be used after plants begin to grow. In the cultivation and in the processing of foods, bacteria make their home in grains and vegetables.

Meat and poultry, because animals eat grain, can contain bacteria like Salmonella, Campylobacter, and Escherichia coli.

Fruits and vegetables and Dairy products can harbor bacteria like Escherichia coli, Salmonella, and Listeria.

Seafood can contain bacteria like Vibrio vulnificus.

Rice as well as other grains contains a bacteria called Bacillus Cereus. Grains should be stored in a cool dry place in sealed containers. They should be checked for signs of spoilage. And one must follow proper cooking and reheating procedures to control the bacteria that lives within.

Foods that contain Bacillus Cereus are Rice, Wheat, Oats, Barley, Corn, Potatoes, Beans, Peas, Other Starchy Vegetables, Dried Herbs and Spices, Dried Fruits and Vegetables, Powdered Milk and other Dried Dairy Products.

The highest risk foods are Rice and Pasta that have been left at room temperature for too long and foods that have not been reheated to a high enough temperature.

To prevent disease from the bacteria in these foods it is necessary to practice proper food handling and storage as well as good hygiene.

We will discuss more about this in the pages to come. In short, be careful with all foods and be willing to enhance your food handling practices. This is not only for your safety but also for your family members and anyone who eats the food prepared in your kitchen.

Practice the admonition – Refrigerate after opening.

The fate of a nation rides on the health of its people.

Chapter 2-Bacillus Cereus

There are several bacteria that are found in foods. Their prevalence changes with areas and cultures because of types of food consumed. I will focus first on B. Cereus and rice. The food handling procedures are the same for all situations. Namely, refrigerate after opening.

B. Cereus is a concern in cooked but unrefrigerated rice. It can produce toxins that cause food poisoning.

When one experiences food poisoning there may be nausea, vomiting, diarrhea, and abdominal cramps. Jesus said, "What goes into the mouth cannot defile the body, because it is eliminated." When the offending poison exits, one feels better immediately. There is usually nothing to worry about. Just stay away from what doesn't agree with your system.

It is not always practical to stay away from the offending bacteria and the toxins it produces because it is part of your life in some cases. It is a cultural thing. So, when you feel better, you go back to eating the same food because that is what is available to you.

Your body then begins building up an immunity to it. The bacteria and the toxins are still there; and they are doing their damage little by little, but your system is used to their presence and doesn't react with the usual symptoms of nausea, vomiting, diarrhea, and abdominal cramps. So, the offending bacteria is not being eliminated. Sometimes it is not in the intestines where it can be eliminated, it is non-intestinal. When it has become a permanent resident of your body, it does whatever damage it will. And just like the boll weevil, this'll be home, my lonely huh huh home. This'll be my home.

Bacillus Cereus originally comes from the earth. The spores are commonly found in soil and can contaminate a variety of foods including rice, vegetables, and dairy products. It contaminates food during cultivation and processing. This came from Meta. I will add that dairy products don't come from the earth directly. They come from cows. Therefore, the cows must be infected with the bacteria first for it to enter the milk from which many products are made. And of course, cows eat grain from which comes the bacteria.

Drinks, cheeses, butter, yogurt, ice cream, as well as other specialized products are made from the milk of cows, sheep, goats, and buffalo. Nothing is dangerous if handled and stored properly. Improper food handling practices can allow B. Cereus to grow and produce toxins.

B. Cereus produces enterotoxins and cereulide, which can cause diarrheal and emetic syndromes. Cereulide is a highly toxic, heat-resistant bacterial toxin that causes severe food poisoning. You could get more than a royal flush. It is a severe health risk and can cause symptoms ranging from nausea and vomiting to acute liver failure and death. The toxin cannot be destroyed by normal cooking temperatures once it has formed. And it comes from Bacillus Cereus which contaminates starchy foods like pasta and rice when improperly handled and stored.

Bacillus Cereus-produced toxins can cause food poisoning that leads to more severe health issues.

Regularly eating contaminated rice can lead to accumulated toxins in the body, potentially causing kidney damage or other health problems.

Bacillus Cereus as well as other bacteria can also be found in food supplements. Probiotics, Herbal supplements, and other supplements can be contaminated with harmful bacteria depending on how they are processed.

Contaminated supplements can cause a range of issues from mild gastrointestinal symptoms to more serious infections. This is a mild statement compared to the diseases and death we have already talked about that can be caused by B. Cereus.

The fate of a nation rides on the health of its people.

Chapter 3-B. Cereus Build-up

Bacillus cereus can build up in the body over the years and potentially cause damage. The bacteria can evade the immune system and establish long term, persistent infections within the body, remaining in a dormant or low-activity state for extended periods, according to the National Institutes of Health.

Certain bacterial infections, like tuberculosis, can remain latent for years without causing any symptoms. They can reactivate under certain conditions, such as a weakened immune system, and lead to disease and damage.

Conditions like small bowel bacterial overgrowth involve a buildup of bacteria in the small intestine that can lead to digestive issues, nutrient deficiencies and damage to the intestinal lining over time if left untreated, according to Penn Medicine.

The presence of antibiotic-resistant bacteria within the body can lead to recurrent infections that are harder to treat and can cause escalating problems over time.

In essence, while the body's immune system actively fights off most bacterial invaders, some bacteria can bypass these defenses and establish a persistent or latent presence within the body that can eventually lead to health problems or a sudden flare-up of symptoms and damage years later.

In rare instances B. Cereus infections can be life-threatening, especially for people with weakened immune systems.

Given the seriousness of B. Cereus, it is crucial to prioritize food safety and handling to minimize the chance of infection.

People who have consumed contaminated rice and other contaminated foods all their lives may experience varying health effects. In some countries rice is a very popular and commonly eaten staple food. Staple means that it is a fundamental part of the diet and eaten regularly. To make cooking and food preparation quicker and easier, some people do not refrigerate their rice at all.

Since they have consumed B. Cereus for an extended period, it will not be eliminated from the body by the usual means. It creates toxins and produces diseases. The body is strong, but B. Cereus will accomplish what it was created to do- damage- destruction - the curse of the ground on which we stand.

The fate of a nation rides on the health of its people.

Chapter 4–The Night of the Black-eyed Peas

For dinner one evening, I was eating black-eyed peas. They were served on a bed of rice. They were spiced with the usual seasonings of the African American culture. They were delicious or at least acceptable.

As I was eating, I was also working on my computer, preparing books for publishing and marketing. As a result, the food I was eating was getting consumed very slowly and in spurts. Some of it was allowed to set for an hour or more.

Something very strange happened. The food began to take on the unmistakable odor of spoilage. I asked myself, "How did I eat all that without noticing that it smelled bad?"

I sat there working for some time longer and the smell increased tremendously. When I was ready to retire for the evening, the smell was so strong that I couldn't stand sitting next to it. I dreaded the task but felt that it was my solemn duty to report the bad food to the cook so she would know not to serve any more of it. I certainly didn't want anyone getting sick over a malady I failed to report. I did that as gently as I knew how, choosing my words carefully.

It backfired! This was a very sensitive cook. I understand better now her allegiance to her culture. But I have feelings too. I am very capable of determining when food is bad and should not be eaten. My whiffer is intact. I am also very capable of knowing when an unpleasant or dangerous situation needs to be reported. I suffered the consequences for days.

Within those days of agony and misery, I had a dream. In the dream I was told, "It was not the black-eyed peas."

Darn, I knew I should have cleaned my moustache.

I was also told in the dream that it was the rice that caused the smell and that rice is the cause, or perhaps only the contributor, of the sarcoid palsy this cook suffers. And the cure or alleviation of the symptoms is to enhance her food handling practices as well as taking the necessary steps to get rid of the B. Cereus and its toxins in her body.

I was very surprised to be given information about another person. I believe that God talks to me about me and to you about you. But it was about me also. I have Multiple Sclerosis, and it has been exacerbated lately, and my walk is not so graceful and I am much more out of balance than usual.

I now realize that it is possible that improper food handling practices have been affecting my health for years. I leave meats and pasta and rice out of the refrigerator overnight and all the next day before I eat it.

Now I have entered a situation where it could be affecting me even more. But also, a loving family is in danger who still eat this food from time to time and have been consuming it for the early years of their lifetime.

And the cook? The decision will be in her hands to change or to remain steadfast in a dangerous situation. Whole cultures can benefit from the research done to put this manuscript together.

It was all because of a meal of black-eyed peas. I would never have known to be serious about B. Cereus had it not been for this experience, the punishment I suffered thereafter, the dream, and the research.

The fate of a nation rides on the health of its people.

Chapter 5-Storing Rice

I wasn't sure what to do about this dream. I will be in much more trouble if I speak against the rice rather than the black-eyed peas. She eats rice every day. And what cook wants to hear that her food handling practices could use some upgrading? But I know that it would be very selfish of me to keep this information to myself. There are lives and well-beings at stake here.

I began researching to find out what could be wrong with the rice. I thought that rice and pasta would still be good for at least a few days when stored out of the refrigerator.

I ask numerous questions of Meta and Gemini. I asked them in different ways to be sure I was getting accurate information. What I learned prompted me to be serious about B. Cereus.

I had been told that after rice is cooked, drained, and dried that it is just like uncooked rice and can be stored indefinitely. So, that was my first question.

Is cooked rice safe to eat when it is stored out of the refrigerator?

Rice that is left out of the refrigerator for more than one hour has already begun to grow spores of bacteria and produce toxins.
Bacillus Cereus is a concern in cooked but unrefrigerated rice because it can produce toxins that cause food poisoning. Here are some reasons to be serious about it:

1. Food poisoning risk: B. cereus can produce emetic (vomiting) and diarrheal toxins, leading to symptoms like nausea, vomiting, diarrhea, and abdominal cramps.

2. Rapid growth: B. cereus can multiply rapidly in cooked rice that's not stored properly, especially in warm temperatures (between 40°F and 140°F).

3. Toxin production: The bacteria can produce toxins that are heat-stable, meaning cooking the rice again might not destroy the toxins.

4. Common contamination source: Cooked rice is a common source of B. cereus contamination, especially if it's left at room temperature for too long.

• • •

To minimize the risk, it's essential to handle cooked rice safely:

Refrigerate cooked rice promptly (within 1-2 hours).

Store it in shallow containers to cool quickly.

Reheat cooked rice to 165°F (74°C) before consumption.

Discard cooked rice that's been left at room temperature for too long (more than 2 hours).
By taking these precautions, you can reduce the risk of B. Cereus contamination and food poisoning.

. . .

On the night of the black-eyed peas, the Bacillus Cereus in the rice was multiplying rapidly at room temperature and producing a bad smell.

The black-eyed peas had been served on a bed of rice which had been stored but not reheated to 165 degrees. The hot juice from the peas was activating and causing rapid growth of the B. Cereus.

. . .

To ensure the safety of cooked rice it is recommended to:

Cool it rapidly after cooking, ideally within one hour.

Store it in a refrigerator at 40 degrees or below in a covered container.

Consume it within 24 hours after cooling and refrigerating.

When reheating, ensure that it is steaming hot throughout, reaching a temperature of 165 degrees.

Never reheat rice more than once.

Awareness of the risks associated with improper cooling and storage is crucial to prevent foodborne illness.

To avoid poisoning from rice, it is crucial to:

Cool and refrigerate cooked rice quickly, ideally within one hour and definitely within two hours.

Store properly, keep cooked rice in airtight containers in the refrigerator.

Reheat thoroughly, ensure reheated rice reaches an internal temperature of at least 165 degrees.

Discard if unsure. If rice exhibits any signs of spoilage (bad smell, slimy texture, discoloration) or has been left at room temperature for too long, it is safest to throw it out, for this is due to bacterial activity.

The fate of a nation rides on the health of its people.

Chapter 6-More About Rice

Cooked and dried rice can be stored safely at room temperature if it is properly dried to a moisture level that is inhospitable to bacterial growth. However, it is crucial to follow safe handling practices.

The drying method must ensure that the rice is dried to a safe moisture level, typically below 10 percent moisture content. The dried rice must be stored in airtight containers to prevent rehydration and contamination. It must be used within a reasonable time frame to ensure quality and safety.

If the rice is not thoroughly dried or is stored in a humid environment, it is better to store it in a refrigerator to prevent bacterial growth, particularly Bacillus Cereus, which can survive cooking and thrive in most environments.

Cooked rice loaded with bacteria will develop a noticeable off or sour smell. Freshly cooked rice should have very little aroma.

Raw rice contains spores of bacteria, Bacillus Cereus, which can survive cooking. If cooked rice is left at room temperature, these spores can germinate and multiply rapidly, producing toxins that can cause food poising.

The toxins produced by Bacillus Cereus and the bacterial metabolism will give the rice a sour or unpleasant smell. It smells like a dirty dish rag. Spoiled rice can become slimy or mushy due to bacterial activity.

• • •

China is the world's largest consumer and producer of rice. It consumes 190,936,000 tons

India is the second-largest consumer, with rice being a staple food for over half its population. It consumes 140,276,000 tons.

Africa is a major consumer of rice and the largest importer of rice.

Asian countries dominate both rice production and consumption, with China and India accounting for over half the world's total rice consumption.

Rice consumption is driven by its cultural significance, affordability, and versatility in diverse cuisines across these nations.

The fate of a nation rides on the health of its people.

Chapter 7-Diseases Caused by Bacillus Cereus

While Bacillus Cereus is primarily known for causing food poisoning with symptoms like nausea, vomiting, diarrhea, and abdominal cramps it can be associated with serious infections, particularly in immuno-compromised individuals- according to the National Institute of Health. In some cases, severe infections can involve the central nervous system and potentially impact facial muscles.

Specifically, there have been reports of Bacillus Cereus causing cranial nerve palsy, which can affect the facial nerve (seventh cranial nerve) and lead to facial weakness or paralysis. However, these instances are rare and usually occur in individuals with weakened immune systems, like patients undergoing chemotherapy for leukemia.

It is important to differentiate this from more common causes of facial paralysis, such as Bell's palsy, which is often linked to viral infections and is more prevalent in the general population.

Therefore, while Bacillus Cereus infection causing issues with facial muscles is uncommon, it can occur in susceptible individuals, particularly those who are immuno-compromised and develop severe infections involving the central nervous system.

Many people with whom I am familiar, including me, can't walk gracefully anymore.

A serious non-intestinal infection by Bacillus Cereus could potentially cause swelling of the lymph nodes behind the knee, known as popliteal lymphadenopathy. This would occur as part of a severe, localized soft tissue infection in the lower leg or foot.

Here is a breakdown of how this could happen:

B. Cereus beyond the gut: While most known for causing food poisoning, B. Cereus can also cause serious extra-intestinal infections, especially in immunocompromised individuals or following a traumatic injury.

Soft tissue infections: In rare but severe cases, B. Cereus can cause necrotizing (flesh-eating) skin and soft tissue infections in the extremities.

Lymphatic drainage: The popliteal lymph nodes behind the knee drain lymph fluid from the lower leg and foot.

Reactive lymphadenopathy: If a significant bacterial infection occurs in the area drained by these nodes, the immune system response can cause the nodes to swell. This is a normal function of the lymphatic system as it works to fight the infection.

Important considerations:

Rarity: An invasive B. Cereus infection leading to popliteal lymphadenopathy is rare, particularly in otherwise healthy individuals. Most infections from this bacterium are mild and gastrointestinal.

Risk factors: People with diabetes, compromised immune systems, or those who have experienced trauma or a medical procedure in the area are at higher risk for severe B. Cereus infections.

Bacillus Cereus (B. Cereus) is a significant foodborne pathogen, but its prevalence varies globally. Here's a breakdown of its prevalence compared to other bacteria.

Global Prevalence: A systematic review and meta-analysis found that the overall prevalence of B. Cereus in foods was approximately 23.746%. The highest prevalence was reported in cereals and beans, with 41.489% and 44.901%, respectively.

Comparison to Other Bacteria: In Brazil, Salmonella sp. was the most prevalent pathogen in foodborne outbreaks (14.4%), followed by Staphylococcus aureus (7.7%), Escherichia coli (6.5%), and B. Cereus (3.1%).

Regional Variations: The prevalence of B. cereus was highest in the Americas and lowest in Australia. Developing countries tend to have a higher prevalence of B. Cereus than developed countries.

Foodborne Disease: B. Cereus is estimated to cause 1.4% to 12.0% of global foodborne outbreaks. It's the second and third most common causative agent of foodborne diseases in France and Europe, respectively.

Some key foods contaminated with B. cereus include:

Aquatic Products: 25.47% of aquatic products in China were contaminated with B. Cereus.

Rice Products: B. Cereus was found in ready-to-eat rice products in Eastern China.

Dairy Products: B. Cereus was detected in dairy products in China.

Vegetables and Spices: B. Cereus can also contaminate raw vegetables and spices.

• • •

No matter what B. Cereus is known to cause, why not be careful to keep it out of your system? It is a bacterium that produces destructive toxins. It can affect your body in ways that are not even known yet. If you have a disease, with an unknown cause and an unknown cure, who can confidently say that B. Cereus didn't contribute to it?

Enhancing your food handling practices may free you from some of the ailments in your body. It may reduce some of the pain in your life. The choice is yours. Keep treating the symptoms of disease or eliminate a potential cause.

The fate of a nation rides on the health of its people.

Chapter 8-Sarcoidosis and Rosacea

In the dream, remember, I was told that the rice was the cause of the cook's Sarcoid Palsy. The general term is Sarcoidosis. Depending on which part of the body is affected, a sub-name is applied.

The cause of Sarcoidosis is unknown, just like the cause of almost all diseases is unknown. The doctors who can think for themselves and get away from the textbook are the ones who help patients the most. They are the ones who most likely can determine the (unknown) cause of a particular disease. They are probably sworn to stick to a code and never go beyond the text, at least don't do it out loud. A thinking person will apply logic to every situation.

Sarcoidosis can affect various parts of the body, including the nervous system, leading to a range of symptoms. When it affects the nervous system, it is known as neuro-sarcoidosis.

Some of the early symptoms of Sarcoidosis are:

Numbness or tingling: Sensory changes in the face, arms, or legs

Weakness: Muscle weakness, especially in the face, arms, or legs

Pain: Headaches, facial pain, or pain in other areas

Vision problems: Double vision, blurred vision, or loss of vision

Seizures: In some cases, neuro-sarcoidosis can cause seizures

Cognitive changes: Memory loss, confusion, or difficulty concentrating

Balance and coordination issues: Difficulty walking or maintaining balance

Other symptoms of sarcoidosis:

Respiratory symptoms: Coughing, shortness of breath, or chest pain

Skin symptoms: Rashes, lesions, or red bumps on the skin

Eye symptoms: Eye pain, redness, or vision problems

Fatigue: Feeling tired or weak

Weight loss: Unexplained weight loss

If you're experiencing any of these symptoms, it's essential to consult a healthcare professional for proper diagnosis and treatment. They can help determine the best course of action and provide guidance on managing symptoms.

That's what doctors do with their medicine. They manage symptoms. They may never cure a disease. To cure a disease, one must take away the cause. I am convinced that some of the incurable diseases we experience, for which the cause and cure are unknown, have legitimate causes and cures. You can either treat the symptoms with medicine for the rest of your life, or you can dig a little deeper in the well of wellness and determine if there is something you are doing that is causing harm to your body.

Sarcoid palsy is not directly linked to consuming contaminated rice. But look at all the evidence we have uncovered already. Even a child can put a block in the same shaped hole. Sarcoidosis is a condition where inflammatory cells form lumps in various organs, often affecting the lungs, skin, or eyes.

The exact cause of sarcoidosis is unknown, but it is believed to be related to genetic and environmental factors. That means family history may play a role and substances or particles from the environment may trigger the disease. It involves an abnormal immune response.

Remember, Bacillus Cereus comes from the soil. That is environment. People from rice-eating countries and ethnic groups are candidates. That is heredity.

• • •

Sarcoidosis is not contagious. It cannot be transferred from one person to another through direct contact or proximity.

Okay, let's uncover more evidence for this cook's condition.

Sarcoidosis is more common in individuals of African and Northern European descent. African Americans, for example, have higher incidence and prevalence rates of Sarcoidosis compared to white individuals. Didn't they say it was related to genetics? This cook was born and raised in Ghana. They also said it was related to environmental factors. Are Bacillus Cereus spores which came from the soil and are growing in rice, part of the environment?

This is from Gemini: Note that contaminated food can contain harmful microorganisms and chemicals, leading to illnesses. In Africa, poor hygiene, unsafe food handling, and inadequate farming practices contribute to food contamination. That's referring to chemicals in foods from fertilizers and pesticides.

According to an article by the National Institutes of Health, Sarcoidosis is believed to be underreported in many regions, especially in Africa.

Several factors suggest that sarcoidosis does affect people in Ghana. There are some documented cases. But their focus is on other diseases. A large portion of the health budget has been allocated to infectious diseases and HIV/AIDS, potentially limiting resources for other conditions like sarcoidosis.

Ghana's healthcare system, like many in Africa, faces challenges with resources and infrastructure, potentially impacting the recognition and diagnosis of complex conditions like sarcoidosis.

The nonspecific nature of sarcoidosis symptoms can lead to delayed diagnosis or misdiagnosis, especially if a comprehensive approach isn't used.

So, while specific statistics might be lacking, it is likely that people in Ghana do have sarcoidosis, and its prevalence might be higher than currently recognized due to challenges in diagnosis and reporting, according to the National Institutes of Health.

There is no known cure for Sarcoidosis, but the disease often resolves on its own. Some individuals find symptom relief through corticosteroids, immunosuppressants, and other medications prescribed by a doctor to manage inflammation. Healthy lifestyle changes such as a balanced diet, regular exercise, stress management, and avoiding lung irritants can also help manage symptoms and improve overall well-being. In some cases, a lung transplant may be considered for advanced lung damage.

The disease often resolves on its own. But how can it resolve if it is fed with Bacillus Cereus daily?

I am out in my hideout writing this while in the house on the counter is a crockpot of rice left over from yesterday. I covered a full serving bowl of it and put it in the refrigerator last night, but the bulk of it remains, waiting for consumption. Rice here is cooked in large quantities because it is easy to just leave it out and grab it by the handfuls or pour hot juice and vegetables over it for a toxic meal.

There is no known cure for Sarcoidosis; but it tears my heart out to witness the way Bacillus Cereus is consumed here. I have given her all the information, from my research, to which she will listen. And I was informed, under no uncertain terms, that the food handling practices are not going to change. I can smell the bacteria in the rice. B. Cereus is also inhaled. The smell is overwhelming when it combines with heated vegetables and their juices. So much spice is added that it camouflages the odor.

Some will not believe (such nonsense) as that which I write. Their diseases have no known cause or cure. I feel it in my body. I have been diagnosed with Multiple Sclerosis thirty years ago. I have managed it over the years with lifestyle changes and exercise. I don't take medicine unless I must. Since I came here, my walk has changed for the worse and my legs and arm muscles have weakened. I have no doubts as to the cause. I will have to find a doctor who will listen to logic or a way to remove toxins from my body.

I experienced the elimination of spoiled food only once; but I believe my body is full of B. Cereus from my own poor food handling practices. Therefore the B. Cereus will live and grow in me.

Our decisions often affect others as well as ourselves. You can't decide to continue with improper food handling and invite others to eat at your table.

Rosacea

While Bacillus Oleronius is more frequently linked to Rosacea, some studies have identified Bacillus Cereus in patients with Rosacea, particularly those with steroid-induced Rosaceiform Dermatitis. The exact role of B. Cereus is not fully understood, but research suggests that its presence, sometimes in association with Demodex mites, may contribute to the inflammatory process of certain Rosacea subtypes.

Bacillus Cereus has been isolated from Demodex Folliculorum mites in some patients with Rosacea, especially those with topical steroid-induced Rosaceiform Facial Dermatitis.

Like other bacteria implicated in Rosacea, B. Cereus may trigger an immune response that leads to inflammation and the development of bumps and pustules.

Bacillus Oleronius is a more commonly cited Bacillus species in Rosacea research, but B. Cereus is a distinct finding in specific cases.

Ongoing research: The exact role and contribution of B. Cereus to Rosacea are still being investigated, and more studies are needed to clarify its significance and the relationship between different Bacillus species and the disease.

While Bacillus Oleronius is the primary bacterial culprit linked to Rosacea, a specific strain of Bacillus Cereus has been found in patients with a Rosacea-like condition, though its role is less defined. Studies show B. Cereus was isolated from Demodex mites in patients with steroid-induced Rosaceiform Dermatitis, suggesting it can play a role, particularly in certain types of Rosacea.

A 2016 study found Bacillus Cereus in Demodex mites from patients with a condition similar to Rosacea, specifically steroid-induced facial Rosaceiform Dermatitis.

The presence of B. Cereus in these cases, along with other bacteria, suggests it may contribute to the development of some Rosacea symptoms, particularly papules and pustules.

More research is needed to understand the exact role of B. Cereus and its significance in the pathogenesis of Rosacea compared to other implicated bacteria like Bacillus Oleronius.

Bacillus Oleronius, another bacterium found in Demodex mites, has a more established link to Rosacea.

This bacterium produces antigens that can trigger an inflammatory immune response, leading to the symptoms of Rosacea.

The fact that the condition improves with antibiotics that target bacteria, even if they don't kill the mites, supports the theory that bacteria play a key role.

• • •

I am using these two diseases, Sarcoidosis and Rosacea, to show the role of bacteria in the maladies that plague mankind. I chose these two because they are affecting individuals whom I love.

Studies have shown that bacterium of some kind is behind the start and the continuation of many diseases.

Why not take steps to rid your body of bacteria and toxins before it's too late? Why not keep bacteria out by enhancing your food handling practices?

Doctors will only treat the symptoms; and sometimes that reinforces the strength of the bacterial toxins. Get one symptom out of the way to create another.

The fate of a nation rides on the health of its people.

Chapter 9-No Cause No Cure

Here are some diseases where the causes or cures are still unknown:

Diseases with Unknown Causes:

Idiopathic Pulmonary Fibrosis (IPF): A progressive lung disease where the lungs become scarred, leading to breathing difficulties.

Chronic Fatigue Syndrome (CFS)/Myalgic Encephalomyelitis (ME): A condition characterized by severe fatigue that doesn't improve with rest.

Fibromyalgia: Widespread musculoskeletal pain and fatigue.

Sarcoidosis: An inflammatory disease affecting multiple organs, including lungs, skin, and eyes.

Complex Regional Pain Syndrome (CRPS): Chronic pain condition, often affecting an arm or leg after an injury.

Interstitial Cystitis/Bladder Pain Syndrome (IC/BPS): Chronic bladder pain without a clear cause.

Irritable Bowel Syndrome (IBS): Gastrointestinal disorder with symptoms like abdominal pain, bloating, and changes in bowel habits.

Essential Tremor: A neurological disorder causing involuntary shaking.

Restless Legs Syndrome (RLS): Uncontrollable urge to move legs which can include discomfort or aching.

Vitiligo: Skin condition characterized by loss of pigment, resulting in white patches.

Diseases with No Cure:

Alzheimer's Disease: A progressive brain disorder affecting memory, thinking, and behavior.

Parkinson's Disease: Neurological disorder affecting movement, balance, and coordination.

HIV/AIDS: Weakens the immune system, making it harder to fight off infections.

Amyotrophic Lateral Sclerosis (ALS): Progressive neurodegenerative disease affecting nerve cells.

Cystic Fibrosis: Genetic disorder causing thick mucus buildup in lungs and the digestive system.

Multiple Sclerosis (MS): Autoimmune disease affecting the central nervous system.

Lupus: Autoimmune disease-causing inflammation and damage to various body parts.
Diabetes (Type 1 and Type 2): Lifelong conditions requiring management through medication, diet, and exercise.

Huntington's Disease: Genetic disorder causing progressive damage to the brain.

Schizophrenia: Severe mental disorder affecting thoughts, feelings, and behavior

Rare and Mysterious Diseases:

Hypertrichosis (Werewolf Syndrome): Excessive hair growth all over the body

Hutchinson-Gilford Progeria Syndrome: Rare condition causing rapid aging in children

Fibrodysplasia Ossificans Progressiva (FOP): Condition where connective tissues turn into bones

Cotard's Syndrome: Neuropsychiatric disorder where people believe they are dead or missing body parts

Alice in Wonderland Syndrome (AIWS)*: Neurological disorder causing distorted body image and hallucinations

These diseases highlight the complexities and challenges in medical research and treatment. Ongoing research and advancements in science offer hope for better understanding and managing these conditions.

What if you could alleviate the symptoms of the conditions in your body simply by upgrading your food handling practices and reducing the growth of bacteria and the multiplication of toxins? Some doctors would be out of business if they could really cure patients. That is one of the reasons they would ridicule patients for applying logic to their health challenges.

The fate of a nation rides on the health of its people.

Chapter 10-Food Handling Strategies

Foods are processed differently today than in the early years of America when we had no electricity and not much for modern conveniences. They are full of preservatives, but they seem to spoil quicker. They are packaged strongly and securely; sometimes you destroy the contents in the process of getting the package open. They must be kept at certain temperatures, over 135 degrees or under 40 degrees. They must be stored adequately. We depend on the Food and Drug Administration to guide us and keep us from blundering into adverse effects on our health.

Before refrigeration, people used various methods to store food and prevent bacterial growth. They would remove moisture from food such as quick-drying fruits, vegetables, and meats.

Smoke shacks were used to preserve meat and fish, which helped to dehydrate it and add a smoky flavor.

Salt was commonly used to draw out moisture and prevent bacterial growth.

Pickling, or soaking food in a solution of brine or vinegar was used to create an acidic environment that inhibited bacterial growth.

Fermenting was used to allow food to break down naturally by microorganisms, which created lactic acid and preserved the food.

Curing with a combination of salt, sugar, and other ingredients was used to preserve meat.

Root cellars, where it was cool and dark with good ventilation were an effective means of storing food to keep it fresh for long periods.

Ice houses, insulated structures, were built and ice was harvested from lakes and rivers to keep food cool.

Cellars and pantries were built into most houses for storing food in cool, dark places to slow down bacterial growth.

These traditional methods are still used today, often in combination with modern preservation techniques, to extend the shelf life of food and prevent spoilage.

Modern technology has given us less time-consuming methods of food preservation. But it may be necessary in some cases to update our food handling practices to prevent bacterial growth and the everyday sicknesses that plague human existence. Perhaps we can even prevent some incurable diseases with unknown causes.

In this book we will focus on the storage and use of cooked and reheated foods. Food, especially after it has been cooked, carries powerful bacteria that can produce toxins that are out to get under your skin and destroy your good health. Some bacteria can even bring about premature death.

• • •

Modern food safety guidelines

For fast food as well as home cooked, there is a two-hour rule. Refrigerate perishable foods, including cooked fish and fries from Long John Silver's, within two hours of cooking.

If the ambient temperature is above 90°F, the time limit is reduced to just one hour. The one-hour rule applies in warmer climate conditions.

This is very important because bacteria that cause food poisoning can multiply rapidly in the "danger zone" between 40 degrees Fahrenheit and 140 degrees Farenheit.

It is best to refrigerate leftovers promptly after the meal to ensure they remain safe to eat later.

Cooked rice

Cooked rice should be cooled and refrigerated as quickly as possible. Even if it came from Dragon Express Chinese Cuisine, rice along with pasta and vegetables must be refrigerated as soon as possible. The two and one-hour limits do not change.

Food storage is for a limited time only. It will only last for about three to four days in the refrigerator.

When reheating, make sure it is steaming hot all the way through to kill any bacteria. It must reach 165 degrees, or the bacteria will thrive.

Do not leave it out for convenience. Never leave cooked rice at room temperature for extended periods as this can lead to the formation of harmful bacteria.

Uncooked rice

Uncooked rice can be stored in a cool, dry place. A pantry is a suitable place to store uncooked rice if it is in an airtight container. This protects the rice from moisture, dust, and pests.

White rice can last for years in a pantry, while brown rice has a shorter shelf life of about six months due to its higher oil content.

The refrigerator or freezer is an option for longer-term storage and to extend shelf life of uncooked rice.

Jams and Jellies

Opened jars of jam and jelly should be refrigerated to prevent spoilage from mold and yeast growth. Unopened jars can be stored at room temperature, refrigerating them after opening is recommended by manufacturers to maintain freshness and flavor, and to extend shelf life significantly. Low-sugar or sugar-free varieties must be refrigerated immediately after opening, as they lack sufficient sugar to act as a preservative.

Refrigeration is necessary after opening to prevent microbial growth. Opening the jar introduces oxygen, and frequent use can introduce contaminants, allowing mold and yeast to grow more quickly. Refrigeration slows down this spoilage process.

Refrigeration can keep open jams and jelly good for six months to a year, whereas they may only last a month or so at room temperature.

Storing in the refrigerator preserves the product's freshness and flavor, maintaining the quality of your purchase.

Always use a clean knife or spoon to avoid introducing bacteria into the jar. That is, wipe the butter or peanut butter off the knife or spoon before dipping it into the jelly.

Storing it in a stable temperature produces best results. In other words, store jars away from the refrigerator door where temperatures fluctuate more.

If you notice signs of spoilage such as a fermented odor, foamy liquid, or mold, discard the product immediately. Don’t take a chance with the health of your family or yourself.

Refrigerate low sugar options immediately. Jams and jellies with reduced or no sugar should be refrigerated from the start.

Sugar is a preservative when large quantities of it are applied. Therefore, syrup can be safely kept out of the refrigerator. It contains two cups sugar to one cup water.

Butter and Margerine

You can store salted butter at room temperature for a few days, but margarine and unsalted butter should be refrigerated. To keep room-temperature butter fresh, store it in a cool place, away from direct sunlight, and in an airtight container or a butter crock to protect it from air and light.

You can keep salted butter on the counter for one or two days, and in some cases, up to three weeks, especially if it is kept in a proper container. The salt acts as a preservative, which inhibits bacterial growth.

Use a butter dish or a butter crock to keep it covered from air and light. If your kitchen is consistently above 70 degrees Fahrenheit, it's safer to keep butter in the refrigerator.

Storing margarine and unsalted butter

Always refrigerate margarine as it typically contains more water and oil, making it more susceptible to bacterial growth and separation at room temperature.

Unsalted butter should be stored in the refrigerator. It does not have salt as a preservative.

General tips

Only leave out as much butter as you can use in a couple of days to prevent spoilage.

Always use a clean utensil to take butter from the container to avoid introducing germs.

Mayonnaise and other condiments

You should not eat mayonnaise that has turned yellow because that is a sign of spoilage. Also, a sour smell, a lumpy texture, or mold indicates bacterial growth. Mayonnaise that has changed color to yellow or brown, regardless of its best-by date, should be discarded.

Yellowing of the mayonnaise can be a sign of chemical breakdown, specifically oil oxidation or rancidity, which makes the mayonnaise unsafe to eat.

This color change is often accompanied by other signs of spoilage, such as an acidic or "stinky" smell, a lumpy or broken-up texture, or the presence of mold.

Throw out any mayonnaise that shows signs of spoilage to avoid potential foodborne illness.

To help prevent spoilage, always keep open mayonnaise refrigerated and check it for spoilage signs before using it. Refrigerate after opening.

Unopened packets of ketchup, mayonnaise, and mustard can be stored out of the refrigerator in a cool, dry place.

Once opened, mayonnaise packets should be refrigerated and used promptly, while ketchup and mustard packets can last slightly longer but are best refrigerated after opening.

Unopened packets can be stored in a cool, dry, dark place: A kitchen drawer or pantry is ideal.

Do not store them in a hot car.

Before using, inspect the packet for any puffiness, tears, or discoloration.

Opened packets of Mayonnaise should be refrigerated immediately and used within a day or two.

Ketchup and mustard can last longer after opening than mayonnaise, but refrigeration is recommended to maintain freshness and quality.

Discard any packet with an odd color, odor, or texture, as these can indicate spoilage.

The low pH from ingredients like vinegar and high sugar content in ketchup and mustard make them shelf-stable before opening.

The packets are sterilized and sealed, preventing contamination until they are opened.

Bread and Multi-grain Bread

Multi-grain bread and other store-bought breads can be stored at room temperature for about five to seven days, but freezing is best for longer storage to prevent it from becoming stale. Refrigeration is generally discouraged as it makes bread become stale faster.

Store bread in a cool, dry place, away from direct sunlight, and in an airtight container, bread box, or the plastic bag it came in. This prevents excessive moisture loss that causes it to become stale and slows down mold growth, which is accelerated by heat and moisture. It will stay fresh for three to five days for homemade bread and five to seven days for commercially prepared bread.

Freezing is used for longer storage.

Tightly wrap sliced or whole loaves in plastic wrap or foil or place them in a freezer-safe bag to prevent freezer burn. Freezing halts the retrogradation process (starch recrystallization), which causes it to become stale, and preserves the quality for months.

Refrigerators are dry environments that speed up the process of losing its freshness, making bread stale and as hard as rubber faster than at room temperature. The drying effect of the fridge also promotes mold growth in certain conditions.

The fate of a nation rides on the health of its people.

Chapter 11-Bacteria Breeding Grounds

Brewed coffee can grow various types of bacteria. Many people will leave coffee in the coffee maker overnight and turn it on in the morning to warm it up. The improperly stored coffee will grow potentially harmful strains of bacteria like Pseudomonas, Staphylococcus, Streptococcus, and E. coli. The specific bacteria that grow depend on the environment, but the risk is higher in warm, moist areas or when brewed coffee is left standing for too long.

Pseudomonas is one of the most prevalent bacteria found in coffee machines, and it can break down caffeine.

Staphylococcus and Streptococcus are Gram-positive bacteria that are often found in coffee makers, according to some studies.

Bacillus is a common gram-positive bacterium, and the predominant genus found in some natural coffee fermentation studies.

Some studies have found E. coli in coffee machines, which is a type of enteric bacteria and can cause fecal contamination.

Klebsiella and Erwinia are common genera found in the microflora during coffee bean fermentation.

The warm, moist conditions in coffee makers provide an ideal breeding ground for bacteria. Bacteria can grow in water reservoirs, spouts, and waste trays.

Once brewed, coffee is no longer sterile. If left at room temperature, it is subject to contamination from the environment and will begin to develop bacteria and mold in 12 to 24 hours. With milk or cream, it is safe for only 2 hours. But what if the coffee maker wasn't cleaned between brews? Then it is already growing bacteria.

While cold brew has a lower risk of bacterial growth, it is not immune. If contaminated ingredients or equipment are used, bacteria can still grow.

You can reduce bacterial growth by cleaning your coffee maker regularly.

Filtered water can help reduce the amount of minerals and bacteria that can build up in your machine.

Wash your coffee cup thoroughly after each use.

Store coffee grounds in an airtight container in a cool, dark place. Do not leave brewed coffee standing out for more than a few hours.

When coffee is left in the pot overnight, it loses flavor due to oxidation and can become stale. While black coffee is generally safe to drink for up to 24 hours at room temperature, its taste deteriorates significantly after just 30 minutes. Coffee with milk or cream should be discarded sooner, ideally within a couple of hours, due to bacterial growth.

Oxidation causes the aromatic compounds in the coffee to break down, leading to a stale and unappealing taste.

Carbon dioxide from the air can dissolve into the coffee, increasing its bitterness.

Bacteria from the environment can grow in coffee, especially if it contains milk or cream. This is particularly true for coffee left at room temperature.

In humid conditions, mold can eventually develop on the coffee over a longer period.

For the best quality, it's recommended to drink coffee shortly after it's brewed.

If you want to save it, refrigerate black coffee in an airtight container. It can last for 3–4 days in the fridge, though the flavor will still decline over time.

Coffee with milk or cream should be discarded after a few hours at room temperature or kept for only one to two days in the refrigerator.

• • •

Food spills and specs in a car can provide an environment for the growth of Bacillus Cereus. B. Cereus is a ubiquitous, spore-forming bacterium found in the environment (soil, dust, etc.) and is a common contaminant of various foods, particularly starchy items like rice, pasta, and potatoes.

B. Cereus spores are commonly tracked into cars on shoes or pets' feet, making their presence highly likely.

Spilled food and specs provide the necessary nutrients for the bacteria to grow.

A car's interior temperature can easily rise to 104°F, when parked. These temperatures are ideal for the spores to germinate (turn into active bacteria) and multiply to hazardous levels.

Once the bacteria multiply to sufficient levels in the food spills or specks, they can produce toxins that cause poisoning when inhaled. These toxins are extremely heat stable and are not destroyed by normal cleaning.

Prevention involves good hygiene and cleaning practices. Clean up all food and drink spills immediately and thoroughly.

Use disinfectants to clean affected areas.

Avoid spills by not eating or drinking in the car. A car is trashed out one speck at a time.

Bacillus Cereus can grow in bacon when spores survive cooking. B. Cereus can form heat-resistant spores that survive the initial cooking process of bacon. These spores will multiply if the cooked bacon is left in the temperature "danger zone" (40°F to 140°F) for an extended period. The spores will germinate and grow into active bacteria. The bacteria multiply and produce toxins that cause food poisoning.

Rapid cooling of cooked food is essential to prevent the spores from germinating and multiplying to dangerous levels.

How to prevent B. cereus in bacon

Cook bacon completely, never partially cook it and save it for later. Keep cooked bacon at temperatures above 140°F if it will be served hot.

Refrigerate any leftovers promptly. The U.S. Food and Drug Administration recommends cooling foods rapidly to prevent the growth of B. Cereus

Storing bacon outside the refrigerator for more than two hours can allow bacteria to grow to dangerous levels, especially for raw bacon. While some dry-cured bacon can last longer at room temperature, most supermarket bacon is not shelf-stable and becomes unsafe to eat due to spoilage signs like a slimy texture, sour odor, or mold.

Raw bacon can be left out for up to two hours, but it must be refrigerated afterward.

After 2 hours throw it away. Perishable foods, including raw bacon, should not be left in the "danger zone" (40°F–140°F) for more than two hours, as harmful bacteria like Salmonella can multiply rapidly.

It's best to refrigerate cooked bacon within two hours. After 2 hours the risk of bacteria growing increases, and the bacon may become slimy, smell sour, or show signs of mold. Cooked bacon can be safely frozen and will last for two to three months.

Bacon is spoiled when you see greenish, grayish, or moldy spots. It will have a sour or sulfuric odor. If the bacon feels slimy, it is a sign of spoilage.

Store unopened bacon in the refrigerator for up to one month. After opening it, wrap it tightly and use it within a week, or freeze it for longer storage. Wrap open bacon tightly in plastic wrap followed by aluminum foil and freeze it. It will last for up to four months.

Bacteria like Staphylococcus aureus, Salmonella, E. coli, and Clostridium perfringens can grow to dangerous levels on bacon if it is left in the "Danger Zone" (40°F–140°F) for too long. While bacon is cured, the salt doesn't always kill these bacteria, especially if it is not cooked thoroughly or is allowed to sit out after cooking.

Staphylococcus aureus is a bacterium that can grow on bacon even with curing salts and cause food poisoning.

Salmonella is a common foodborne pathogen found in raw meat and poultry that can grow on bacon if it's not cooked to a safe temperature.

Another is a general pathogen called E. coli. It can multiply in the "Danger Zone" and lead to illness.

Clostridium perfringens is a bacteria that is commonly found on raw meat and poultry and will grow in large batches of food that are held at unsafe temperatures.

Listeria monocytogenes will contaminate raw meat and is a risk in bacon that is not properly cooked.

Yersinia can also be found in pork products and is a risk if bacon is not cooked thoroughly.

Stay safe by cooking bacon thoroughly. Ensure the bacon is cooked until it is crispy and not chewy to kill potential bacteria and parasites like Trichinella.

Keep hot food hot and cold food cold. If you are serving hot bacon, keep it in a warm place at or above 140°F.

Don't leave cooked bacon out for more than two hours. Refrigerate any leftovers within that time frame.

Never eat raw bacon, as it poses a significant risk of foodborne illness.

These are only a few places where bacteria can grow. There are many more. We will be enhancing our food handling practices if we use good hygiene, that is, keep it clean. When we keep our hands clean and our workplace clean, bacteria will vanish. When we use and store food at safe temperatures, there will be no risk of foodborne illness.

If you take the apathetic position that it doesn't matter, you have lived all these years and you are still alive and healthy, you could be making a mistake. Praise the Lord for your good health but be mindful of those around you. They may be suffering in silence because of your poor decisions. And your time could be at hand.

The fate of a nation rides on the health of its people.

Chapter 12-Healing Strategies

Bacteria and the toxins they create are starters and fuel for many diseases. Why not turn the ignition off by taking steps to detox your body. Bacillus Cereus shows up everywhere, reeking destruction in bodies. Don't blame the bacterium. It must do what it was designed for. It has no choice but to perform as it was programmed. But you have choices. You have the power to make things happen. You can design a healing strategy that will make you whole and healthy again or keep you that way.

Doctors treat symptoms by prescribing medications. That is what they know how to do.

Here are some symptoms that indicate a severe Bacillus infection. B. Cereus infections go beyond typical food poisoning and often suggest the bacteria have spread into the bloodstream or other tissues (septicemia). The specific symptoms depend on the type of infection (B. cereus vs. B. anthracis) and the affected body system.

Regardless of the specific Bacillus species, if the infection becomes systemic (sepsis), symptoms can be life-threatening and require immediate medical attention:

High fever and chills

Rapid heart rate (tachycardia)

Rapid breathing or shortness of breath

Low blood pressure (hypotension)

Confusion, disorientation, or altered mental state

Extreme pain or discomfort

Extreme tiredness or fatigue

Signs of organ dysfunction, such as decreased urine production or abdominal swelling

While B. cereus is known for self-limiting food poisoning, severe non-intestinal infections can occur, particularly in immunocompromised individuals:

Endophthalmitis (severe eye infection): Intense eye pain, a red eye, low vision, and potentially a ring-shaped corneal ulcer. This can lead to permanent vision loss or eye removal if not treated quickly.

Meningitis (brain and spinal cord inflammation): Severe headache, stiff neck, fever, confusion, and possibly convulsions.

Bacteremia/Septicemia: Fever, chills, fatigue, and potential involvement of other organs, such as endocarditis (heart valve infection).

Gangrene: Severe pain, swelling, and tissue death around a wound site.

Anthrax symptoms depend on the route of exposure and can rapidly become severe in the systemic phase:

Inhalational Anthrax: Initial flu-like symptoms (cough, mild fever, body aches) are followed by rapid, severe breathing problems, chest discomfort, drenching sweats, and shock. A chest X-ray may show characteristic widening of the mediastinum (chest area).

Gastrointestinal Anthrax: Severe abdominal pain, bloody vomiting, bloody diarrhea, sore throat, painful swallowing, and swelling of the neck or abdomen.

Cutaneous Anthrax: A painless skin sore with a black center (eschar) that develops from a small, itchy bump. While often localized, extensive swelling may cause difficulty breathing if located on the neck or face, or it can progress to fatal septicemia if untreated.

Injection Anthrax: A deep infection or abscess at the injection site, potentially with fever and chills, which can progress quickly to systemic illness.

If any of these severe symptoms are present, particularly in someone with a weakened immune system, recent trauma, or potential anthrax exposure, seek emergency medical care immediately

Medical Treatment

Serious Bacillus infections are typically treated with intravenous antibiotics such as vancomycin, ciprofloxacin, gentamicin, or imipenem, often in combination. The specific medications depend heavily on the Bacillus species involved (e.g., B. anthracis vs. B. cereus) and the severity and location of the infection.

B. Cereus is notably resistant to common beta-lactam antibiotics (like penicillin and most cephalosporins) because it produces beta-lactamases.

Vancomycin is generally the drug of choice for severe B. cereus systemic infections.

In cases of severe systemic infections, such as meningitis, a combination of vancomycin and an aminoglycoside (like gentamicin) may be used.

Other effective antibiotics include imipenem, chloramphenicol, and clindamycin (though resistance to clindamycin can vary).

For localized infections like abscesses or severe eye infections (endophthalmitis), surgical debridement or drainage is often necessary in addition to antibiotics.

B. anthracis, the cause of anthrax, is generally susceptible to penicillin, but because of potential bioterrorism concerns involving resistant strains, treatment guidelines often recommend specific broad-spectrum agents.

Ciprofloxacin or doxycycline are the primary recommended antibiotics for both treatment and post-exposure prophylaxis, particularly in bioterrorism-related cases.

Serious, systemic anthrax infections (such as inhalational anthrax or meningitis) require combination therapy with multiple intravenous drugs. A common regimen includes a bactericidal agent (e.g., ciprofloxacin or meropenem) plus a protein synthesis inhibitor (e.g., clindamycin or linezolid).

In severe cases, antitoxins (like raxibacumab or obiltoxaximab) may be administered as an adjunct to antibiotic therapy to neutralize the bacterial toxins.

Antibiotic resistance testing is crucial to guide definitive therapy, as susceptibility patterns can vary.

Food poisoning caused by B. cereus is usually self-limiting and does not require antibiotic treatment; supportive care (rest and fluid replacement) is sufficient.

Early treatment is vital for serious infections to improve outcomes and reduce mortality.

RICE is an acronym that helps clinicians remember some of the treatment options for food poisoning/infection caused by B. cereus. Treatment includes rest, intravenous antibiotics for severe infections, cool compresses for fevers, and electrolyte replacement to prevent dehydration.

Health and Wellness

Health and Wellness Technicians do not treat specific diseases. They work to promote wellness throughout the body. In this case where I know my body is full of B. Cereus toxins as well as others, I investigate Detox Strategies. The body has its own ways of detoxification, but when it is overwhelmed with toxins because Bacillus Cereus has become its constant companion, it may need some extra boost by a knowledgeable technician.

Colon Flush

The first thing I tried was a Colonic because I wanted to reduce the methane gas I was expelling, and I wanted to get intestinal toxins out.

A lubricated tube is gently inserted into the anus and up into the rectum. Through the tube a large volume of water, which can be mixed with coffee, runs into the colon to flush it out. Waste, and anything the body will release, is washed out past the small tube and into the waste elimination system. You are in a lying position with your legs up. It is comfortable and minimally invasive. It feels good to be flushed out, unlike a doctor's royal flush for a colonoscopy.

Foot Detox

I needed non-intestinal toxins removed also so I did the Foot Detox. You place your feet in a pan of water which is attached to an electronic device to churn the water and stimulate the removal of toxins. The water changes color with the results.

Gemini criticizes the foot detox as well as the colonic. But that is only doctors against wellness speaking.

My legs function a little better after detox. It will take some repeated treatments to get it out.

Lymph Massage

Lymph node drainage is effective for managing specific conditions, particularly lymphedema, by reducing fluid buildup, swelling, and related symptoms like fatigue and pain. It is performed as a specialized massage or as part of a comprehensive treatment plan. However, it may not be suitable for everyone, and it is crucial to consult a doctor to determine if it's appropriate and to perform it correctly, as some people with heart conditions, infections, or certain other issues should avoid it.

Lymphatic drainage massage stimulates the lymphatic system to increase its capacity to process and move fluid.

This helps to filter out waste products, dead cells, and excess proteins from tissues that have accumulated due to swelling.

It can also increase the production of lymphocytes, which can help the body fight infection.

It is often a key component in managing both primary (congenital) and secondary (caused by cancer treatment, injury) lymphedema.

It can alleviate swelling and feelings of fullness that occur after cancer treatment.

It may help with certain conditions that cause inflammation or swelling, such as arthritis.

Manual lymphatic drainage can be used to aid in exercise recovery.

It is essential to talk to a healthcare provider before starting any lymphatic drainage therapy, especially if you have a pre-existing condition.

Lymphatic drainage massage may not be suitable for individuals with conditions such as active cellulitis, deep vein thrombosis, heart conditions, or certain infections.

It is primarily a way to manage symptoms and improve quality of life, not a cure for the underlying conditions.

For effective and safe treatment, it should be performed by a trained and certified manual lymphatic drainage therapist. They can also teach you self-massage techniques to use at home if appropriate.

For lymphedema, lymphatic drainage is often most effective when used as part of a comprehensive treatment plan, such as Complete Decongestive Therapy (CDT), rather than on its own.

When I did the Lymph Massage, restless leg syndrome activated in my right foot and ankle. There were 5 or 6 painful spasms and then it deactivated. So that tells me that it is doing something. Afterwards, I did a colonic to remove lymphatic fluid. It worked! I viewed the results of what came out. So, that is a good way to remove some toxins.

Lymphatic vessels collect excess fluid, cellular waste, and toxins that have accumulated in the interstitial spaces between cells. This fluid, known as Lymph, is then filtered through the Lymph Nodes where specialized immune cells help to identify and eliminate pathogens, toxins, and other harmful substances.

Biofeedback

For situations involving B. Cereus that have progressed to disabilities in the body, biofeedback is an option for overcoming some disfunctions.

Standard biofeedback uses sensors to monitor the body's electrical activity, such as muscle or brain signals, and translates that information into feedback like sounds or visuals. Some specialized biofeedback therapies, like certain types of electrical stimulation biofeedback, do use electrical impulses for therapeutic purposes, often to help with muscle re-education or pain relief.

Sensors are placed on the skin to measure involuntary bodily functions like heart rate, muscle activity (EMG), or sweat gland activity.

The machine translates these electrical signals into real-time feedback, helping you become aware of them.

With training, you learn to consciously control these functions, such as relaxing your muscles or slowing your heart rate.

The sensors are only measuring the electrical signals your body is already producing, not sending them in.

There is Biofeedback with electrical stimulation. This is a specific type of therapy that combines biofeedback with electrical stimulation.

It uses a small electrical current to help a patient learn to control or relax specific muscles, or to suppress unwanted movements, as in the case of bruxism (jaw clenching).

The goal is to retrain muscles or alleviate pain by using the electrical impulses in conjunction with the biofeedback to create a desired response.

Biofeedback teaches you to control bodily functions like heart rate and muscle tension to reduce stress and manage health conditions. By using sensors to provide real-time feedback on these responses, it helps you learn to consciously alter them, which can lead to improved health outcomes for issues like headaches, incontinence, and stroke recovery. It is a non-invasive learning tool that promotes self-regulation, and the skills learned can be practiced even without the device.

It measures bodily signals, sensors are placed on the body to measure physiological responses such as heart rate, breathing, muscle tension, skin temperature, or brainwave activity.

It provides real-time feedback. This information is converted into a visual or auditory signal (like a changing light or sound) that you can see or hear in real-time.

It teaches self-regulation. You learn to use this feedback to consciously change your physiological responses. For example, when you are stressed, your heart rate might increase; biofeedback helps you learn how to consciously slow it down.

With practice, these self-regulation skills are internalized, and you can control these functions automatically without the device.

By learning to control heart rate and breathing, it can lower overall stress and anxiety levels.

It has shown a positive effect on reducing the frequency and severity of migraines and tension-type headaches.

It can help people regain muscle function after a stroke or spinal cord injury and can strengthen pelvic floor muscles for those with incontinence.

It can help people regain control over bowel and bladder movements by improving muscle strength and rectal sensation.

It can help manage chronic pain by teaching you to control your body's reaction to painful stimuli.

While not as effective as medication, biofeedback may help lower blood pressure slightly.

It serves as a skill-training tool to help regain the use of limbs after a stroke

Biofeedback can help manage multiple sclerosis (MS) symptoms by improving muscle control, reducing pain and fatigue, and helping with bladder and bowel control. Electromyographic (EMG) biofeedback can improve muscle strength and function, especially when combined with exercise, and other forms can help reduce stress, anxiety, and sleep problems.

EMG biofeedback uses sensors to monitor muscle activity, providing real-time feedback to help patients learn to use muscles correctly. Studies show this can lead to improved muscle strength, better walking ability, and enhanced knee function.

Pain management: By helping to relax muscles and reduce tension, biofeedback can be a useful tool for managing MS-related pain, such as migraines, tension headaches, and lower back pain.

Studies have shown that biofeedback can help reduce anxiety, fatigue, and stress in people with MS.

Biofeedback can help with urinary incontinence and bowel incontinence by training the muscles involved in these functions. It can be a useful complement to pelvic exercises for those who have difficulty isolating the correct muscles.

Some research suggests that biofeedback, including vibrotactile biofeedback, may help improve balance control.

Biofeedback techniques can also help with other psychological symptoms like anxiety, depression, and insomnia that can accompany MS.

Biofeedback is considered a complementary therapy, meaning it works best alongside other treatments and therapies, not as a replacement for them.

While promising, more research is needed to fully understand the long-term effects of biofeedback for MS.

Some studies on specific symptoms, like urinary incontinence, have had mixed results.

It is important to discuss biofeedback with a healthcare provider to see if it is a suitable option for your specific situation and to find a qualified practitioner.

Biofeedback can help with hearing loss, particularly by addressing associated symptoms like tinnitus and by providing tools for speech training. While not a direct cure for hearing loss itself, it can improve quality of life by managing the stress and perception of tinnitus and helping individuals with hearing loss learn to produce clearer speech.

Biofeedback can help people learn to control the physiological responses associated with stress, which in turn can reduce the perception and annoyance of tinnitus. Some studies have shown that biofeedback can lead to significant improvements in tinnitus symptoms.

For individuals who are deaf or hard of hearing, spectrographic biofeedback can be used as a training tool to improve speech production. This visual-acoustic biofeedback shows the user how their speech sounds, helping them adjust and refine their pronunciation of consonants and vowels.

Biofeedback teaches patients to control involuntary body functions like pulse and muscle tension, leading to stress reduction. Since stress can exacerbate tinnitus, this can lead to a reduction in symptoms.

Biofeedback does not restore lost hearing. It is a complementary therapy that addresses the effects of hearing loss.

Focus on associated symptoms: The primary benefit of biofeedback is in managing the stress, anxiety, and perception of tinnitus that often accompany hearing loss.

It is best to consult with a professional to determine if biofeedback is the right approach for your specific needs.

Biofeedback and related techniques like neurofeedback and cognitive brain training can potentially help with some hearing-related issues where the problem is in the brain, such as difficulty understanding speech in noise or tinnitus. These methods train the brain to process auditory information more effectively and manage symptoms, but they cannot stimulate activity in the brainstem and are not a substitute for medical advice or treatment for hearing loss that stems from the ear itself.

Neurofeedback is a type of biofeedback that uses real-time displays of brainwave activity to teach self-regulation.

It can help with conditions like tinnitus by teaching the brain to divert attention away from the perceived sound.

It may help with sensory integration and auditory processing issues by influencing brainwave activity.

Cognitive brain training involves specific exercises, sometimes using games, to improve cognitive function and the brain's ability to process sound.

It can help people, especially older adults, become "sharper" and better at picking out speech in noisy environments.

Some studies have shown that playing certain video games can improve the ability to understand speech in noisy settings.

Auditory training can help retrain the brain to better process sound once hearing is restored through other means, such as hearing aids.

It helps the brain learn to distinguish between sounds more clearly.

It can improve listening stamina by reducing the mental effort required to hear.

These methods are generally focused on the brain's processing, not on restoring function to the ear itself. Other types of hearing loss may require different treatments, such as hearing aids or medical intervention.

It is crucial to get a professional diagnosis from an audiologist to determine the root cause of your hearing issues and to get the most appropriate treatment plan.

Biofeedback, neurofeedback, and cognitive training are best used under the guidance of a qualified professional who can determine if they are right for your specific situation.

Biofeedback can help with ED, particularly as part of pelvic floor physical therapy. By using biofeedback to help you learn to control and strengthen your pelvic floor muscles, you can improve erectile function, penile blood flow, and ejaculatory control.

Biofeedback-assisted exercises help improve awareness and control of pelvic floor muscles, which are important for achieving and maintaining an erection.

Studies have shown that biofeedback-guided pelvic floor muscle training can result in greater improvement in erectile function compared to exercises alone.

Some research suggests that biofeedback-assisted exercise interventions may contribute to improved penile blood flow.

Visual and auditory feedback on muscle activity can increase a patient's confidence in their ability to control their muscles during sexual activity.

Biofeedback provides an effective treatment option that doesn't involve medication and has fewer side effects.

The effectiveness of biofeedback can depend on factors like patient compliance and the severity of the dysfunction.

It's important to work with healthcare professionals who can guide a personalized approach to treatment.

Biofeedback is often used alongside other treatments, such as low-intensity pulsed ultrasound (LIPUS), to further improve outcomes.

The cost of biofeedback can vary significantly, with in-office sessions ranging from $50 to $300 per session, while home-use devices offer a more affordable one-time purchase. The total cost depends on factors like the type of biofeedback, the number of sessions required, insurance coverage, and whether you choose professional sessions or an at-home device.

The cost typically ranges from $50 to $300 per session, depending on the provider and location.

Many treatment plans require 10 to 40 sessions for lasting results, which can add up quickly.

Some clinics offer discounts for purchasing multiple sessions upfront.

Coverage varies widely among insurance providers, so it's crucial to check with your insurance company ahead of time.

The can range from $20 to $1,000, with some high-quality devices available for around $200.

A one-time purchase allows for flexible and more affordable training over a long period.

It requires you to be self-motivated and may not include the guidance of a professional.

Neurofeedback sessions often cost more than other types due to more expensive equipment.

Clinics in larger cities or those with highly specialized practitioners may charge higher rates.

Insurance coverage is a major factor, as not all insurance plans cover biofeedback, and coverage can vary by condition.

The total cost is heavily influenced by how many sessions are needed to achieve your goals.

The fate of a nation rides on the health if its people.

Summary

The introduction of this book begins with warm kind words for the men and women who work in the kitchen to cook for their families and themselves. It expresses an understanding of why some things are done out of habit that are not beneficial. It gives encouragement to open the mind of the reader to the need for learning and enhancing our food handling practices.

The introduction clearly states what this book is about and why it is written. It tells what the focus of the book is, a bacterium called Bacillus Cereus, along with the whys and wherefores and pertinent information about B. Cereus. It tells where the 80 pages of information came from and lists a few of the reputable sources.

It expresses hopes for the book to reach certain groups of people. And lastly it makes the profound statement, **The fate of a nation rides on the health of its people.**

Chapter 1 expresses the idea that bacteria make their home in our food. It tells us where bacteria come from and in what foods they can be found. The highest risk foods are rice and pasta that were cooked and left too long at room temperature and then not heated to high enough temperature to kill the bacteria. It begins to introduce the idea that we can prevent the growth of bacteria and prevent the distresses of food-borne illness. It leaves you with the admonition, **refrigerate after opening.**

Chapter 2 introduces Bacillus Cereus. It tells how it creates food poisoning. It tells where it comes from. It tells what foods are contaminated with it. It tells what toxins are created by Bacillus Cereus and what they can do to the body.

Chapter 3 states that Bacillus Cereus can build up in your body over time, evade the immune system, and cause damage years later. It cites some of the serious health effects.

Chapter 4 is the reason the book is being written. An incident happened that caused trouble in a relationship. It opened the door for lots of research and writing, a message that people need to hear for their own safety, and the safety of their families. Pain, destruction, and even death may enter the families of those who will not listen to good sound advice. **It is not a laughing matter, but some people treat it that way.**

Chapter 5 talks about the storing of rice, which is the most dangerous food you can eat when left out of the refrigerator to grow bacteria. It talks about some of the dangers of food poisoning and how to avoid it.

Chapter 6 talks more about rice, and how to identify when the rice is spoiled. It talks about the major rice consuming countries. **The bacteria and toxins from spoiled rice is a worldwide dilemma that most people don't even know about.**

Chapter 7 talks about some of the diseases caused by Bacillus Cereus. It tells of some of the key foods contaminated with B. Cereus. **No matter what the bacteria is known to cause, why not keep it out of your system or take steps to get rid of it if it's already there?**

Chapter 8 describes Sarcoidosis and Rosacea. Bacillus Cereus has been found to be associated with both diseases. **It doesn't matter if this bacterium caused the disease or not, it aggravates the symptoms and causes more destruction in the body of the person who harbors it and grows it.**

Chapter 9 enumerates many of the diseases for which is claimed, it has an unknown cause and an unknown cure. It lists some rare and mysterious diseases. **Enhancing your food handling practices may eliminate some diseases and much of the pain in your body.**

Chapter 10 gives you some food handling practices. It tells of the way food was stored before we had electricity and refrigerators and all the conveniences of today. It lists some of the commonly used foods and gives good handling practices for each.

Chapter 11 gives you some bacteria breeding grounds that we wouldn't even think of. It tells of the various bacteria that could come from these foods.

Chapter 12 gives you the symptoms that indicate a severe Bacillus infection. It lists more of the diseases that Bacillus Cereus can cause. It gives you some healing strategies doctors use for a Bacillus Cereus infection. It gives you some health and wellness strategies to use if your body is already full of bacteria and toxins. You can use doctors and medicine. You can use the body's natural detox system. And you can use health and wellness strategies that aid lymph draining and detoxing.

The fate of a nation rides on the health of its people.

Conclusion

I have come to a conclusion- B. Cereus is something about which to Be Serious. Every day I watch my friend suffer. Mucus pours from her eyes. Often, she holds her head in her hands. But she denies that anything is wrong. She prides herself on being 75 years old and healthier than me at 70. She laughs at my ideas about B. Cereus. She says it has nothing to do with her condition. The cause and the cure are unknown. She takes her pills and supplements. She continues to consume spoiled rice and vegetables. She won't refrigerate her cooked foods promptly. The whole situation rips my heart out, especially when she chops me down for my ideas about food safety. I keep working on me and my legs which developed an ungraceful walk since I came here.

Today I am walking normally. Something is happening. I hope it continues. I use health and wellness and the body's natural detoxification processes. I use exercise instead of visiting a doctor. My friend is a nurse. She pokes insults at me saying, "Those practices thrive on people like you." "Why don't you take care of yourself?" She knows her body, and everything is ok. She takes care of herself.

I suffer in silence. I just hope this information reaches people who can reach her before it is too late. Her children are all in the medical profession. They don't know about any of this. But they have been subjected to it. I would not want one of them to suffer. If B. Cereus did strike, it might be a different ailment. I would be laughed at and punished if I intruded in her family affairs. This is part of the proof that B. Cereus is something about which to Be Serious.

The point is: B. Cereus is a powerful bacterium that creates toxins that destroy a person's health. It can cause disease, or it can aggravate disease that has another cause or an unknown cause. It can be detected in the body, and it can be treated.

Point B is the world is full of toxins. They enter our bodies in various ways. Strong bodies handle them adequately. Sometimes the body needs a little help in handling armies of spores that attack by surprise.

Enhancing your food handling practices can keep B. Cereus out of your body, if it is not already there. Even if you don't know what causes your ailments, detoxing your body and enhancing your food handling practices will be beneficial to your health.

If you don't know something, Google it. Gemini will be happy to help. All this information came from various professional sources through Meta and Gemini.

If you want to get toxins out of your body, there are many sources of help. I will not vouch for any of them. I am still working on me. I do know that I will Be Serious about B. Cereus and enhance my food handling practices.

The fate of a nation rides on the health of its people.

www.ingramcontent.com/pod-product-compliance
Lightning Source LLC
LaVergne TN
LVHW022305200926
848481LV00004B/1224

* 9 7 9 8 2 3 3 3 4 9 2 6 3 *